Natural hair maintenance

How to maintain your natural hair with onion and rice water.

By Philemon Nancy

Table of contents

Introduction

Afro-textured hair, or kinky hair, is the hair texture of populations in Africa. Each strand of this hair type grows in a tiny, angle-like helix shape. The overall effect is such that, contrasted with straight, wavy or curly hair, afro-textured hair appears denser.

In this short book you will learn easy steps in maintaining your natural hair.

- **<u>Skipping Wash day</u>**:

Skipping wash day may be tempting, especially if you're putting on a protective style like box braids, since washing can create curls. But it's healthy to wash your hair every 7 to 10 days in order to keep your scalp healthy. To prevent curls, dilute your normal shampoo and transfer it to a bottle, or try one of several brands that produce shampoos for use while putting on protective styles. Look for products that cleanse the scalp without disrupting your style, such as ApHogee Keratin & Green Tea Shampoo.

- **Steaming your hair**: Steam treatments are popular among people with natural hair, and for good reason. They help revive curls and increase shine and elasticity to the hair by opening up the cuticle to allow in more moisture. I recommend the EZBASICS Hair And

Facial Steamer. For best results, you should steam for 20 to 30 minutes at a time, and do it either in between shampoos or every time you condition your hair. Another tip to get the most out of your steam sessions, do a hot oil treatment at the same time. I recommend Coconut

Oil or almond oil cause they are best known for keeping coily hair moisturized. If you don't have a steamer at home, you have a few options, like using your facial steamer (if you have one of those). Hooded or standing hair dryers can also work to deep-condition the hair in a pinch, but just know that they're not as good as steaming. Steaming is more helpful because it's wet heat instead of dry heat. But if you only have a hooded dryer, that is still a good option for a deeper condition. Before sitting under your hooded dryer, place a plastic cap over your curls to help lock in

moisture while conditioning.

- **Seeking professional help for guidance on protein treatments**: Protein can obviously be helpful here, but it's possible to go overboard, which is why I suggest scheduling a video consultation with your stylist to get the best recommendations for your hair type. Too much protein can be bad because once you have enough, the hair can become too strong and breakable. Aside from an at-home consultation with your hair care mentor, if you opt for a protein treatment, i recommend mixing a moisturizing mask with a protein treatment once a month, so you get the benefits of both.

- **Using leave-in conditioner**: Never underestimate the power of a leave-in conditioner. I recommend using a leave-in conditioner every one to two days to make sure your hair stays moisturized when wearing a protective style. To ensure you don't end up with a white cast or miss any strands, you can mix your leave-in conditioner with water in one continuous spray bottle and aloe vera with water in another bottle, and spray your hair as needed.

- **Sealing your ends**: Dry ends are another daily pain point for many natural hair, but oils and heavy creams are a good solution to help seal the ends. Argan oil is a very moisturizing oil because of its vitamin E content and fatty acids, Jojoba oil is very moisturizing because it contains vitamins A, B, C, and E, and minerals like zinc and copper. I use Jojoba oil and it keeps my ends moisturized without leaving behind an oily remnant. Dry ends can often indicate that it's time for a trim, and you can try that at home if you feel comfortable to. Twist the hair in plats and cut off the thinnest part where the twist ends.

Maintaining your hair with onion and rice water.

People often misuse the procedures in using rice water and onion juice to maintain the hair. In this book, you're going to learn how to do that. Here is another easy yet the best remedy in maintaining your hair. The use of onion and rice water.

Ingredients

Rice

Onion

Water

Procedure

Step 1: Boil rice with enough water for about fifteen minutes (depending on the amount you're making) and allow to cool.

Step 2: Wash the onion and blend with water.

Step 3: Drain out the water from the onion (onion juice).

Step 4: Separate the water from the rice after cooling and add the onion juice to the rice

Steps to apply on the hair

There are two ways in applying the onion and rice water remedy on the hair:

- Before washing method
- After washing method

Before washing method

Step 1: Apply it on your hair and cover with a plastic bag.

Step 2: Leave it for about 30 minutes.

Step 3: Then wash with shampoo (shampoo with mint or tea tree is a good remedy) and rinse.

After washing method

Step 1: Wash your hair thoroughly with a good shampoo and rinse it

Step 2: Apply the onion juice and rice water on your hair and cover with a plastic bag

Step 3: Leave for about 30 minutes and rinse

Step 4: After rinsing, make sure to apply deep conditioner on your hair

(Cantu grapeseed conditioner is a good remedy) and leave for about 15 minutes.

Step 5: After the deep conditioner,rinse again (to avoid hair breakage)

Step 6: Apply leave in conditioner and style your hair (you can use a con crow or you can twist it) and leave until it dry.

Conclusion

I hope with this remedy you'll be able to maintain your natural hair and come back with good reviews.

www.ingramcontent.com/pod-product-compliance
Lightning Source LLC
LaVergne TN
LVHW021353160826
845679LV00008B/1606